Brace Yourself

Surviving adult orthodontia

*Everything your orthodontist
didn't tell you
and some of the things she did*

*How to eat, drink and be merry
despite the metal in your mouth*

*Specific hints, clues and recommendations
for those months (years) you will spend
in braces*

*How to buck up and find the joy
when your mouth is enslaved*

We did it; you can too!

By
Pamela Hobart Carter
and
Lynn Wiley Grant

Please visit our Pinterest page for updated recipes, humor, tips, history, and all things BRACES.

http://www.pinterest.com/pamelahobartcar/brace-yourself/

Table of Contents

Physical and Emotional Changes.
Expectations and Adjusting to Life after
Braces. Face and Mouth. Lifestyle.
Penultimate Chapter. Self-Esteem. Sex.
Smiling. Support. Trauma. Weight.

Eating changes.
Breakfast.
Lunch.
Supper.
Restaurant Dining.
Post-Braces Party Menu.

Why do we do it? Cosmetics and Malocclusion.
Trauma.

Introduction

We decided to write this guide because we were shocked by how much wearing braces caused us to modify our lives. We kept saying to ourselves, *If only I'd known* ... Many of our problems and pitfalls could have been avoided—or softened—if we'd had a dandy little tome like this one.

Why should you read this guide? If you already wear braces, you'll get information that your orthodontist won't give you. This book will help you negotiate orthodontia with less pain and a better sense of what is to come. If you are considering wearing braces, this guide will help you to make informed decisions. If you live with or love someone who is wearing braces, this guide will help you to help them through the experience. If you have clients, colleagues, or patients who wear braces, they will appreciate your new understanding of their trials and tribulations.

Even if you wore braces as a child, you are in for a new experience. Treatment for adults is, by necessity, a compromise and differs from that for a child because the adult's growth is complete ("Orthodontics-A Patient's Education Guide" by the American Association of Orthodontics, Jack Dale). A child's teeth and jaws are more malleable and many complications that are avoidable for children are unavoidable for adults. The whole process is potentially more complex and lengthy than it was for the adolescent. We'll warn you about the differences.

The majority of information about braces comes from orthodontists and while they are the experts on straightening teeth and correcting bites, they are not necessarily experts on the experience of wearing braces.

They will give you opinions based on dental health and on American standards of a "normal" mouth. After all, it is their business. We are interested only in passing information to you that we believe will improve your experience of orthodontia. We hope to make your experience less uncomfortable than our own.

When Edward Hartley Angle developed the idea of orthodontics in a form we can recognize as "modern" in the 19th century, he most probably had dental health and function on his mind. When we launched into the orthodontics ourselves, we had dental health and function and esthetics on our minds. We were outcome-oriented: *"When I'm done with this people will stop asking me why my teeth look squished."* Little did we suspect what the psychological and physical ramifications would be *during* the process.

This is not to say that the braces experience is uniform for all wearers. We talked with many individuals in an effort to give you a full picture of what you may experience and included quotations and anecdotes from these braces wearers. When we say, "Some patients," or "Many braces wearers," we are referring to the individuals with whom we spoke. We thank them for their willingness to share their experiences with us.

Brace yourself for straight information.

Lynn and Pam

Chapter 1

How to Choose an Orthodontist and a Treatment Plan

Orthodontics is the branch of dentistry that specializes in the diagnosis, prevention and treatment of dental and facial irregularities ... [The] practice of orthodontics requires professional skill in design, application and control of corrective appliances [braces] to bring teeth, lips and jaws into proper alignment and achieve facial balance.

(American Association of Orthodontists pamphlet "Facts About Orthodontics")

Finding the Right Orthodontist

Finding the right orthodontist is key. Start by asking your dentist. She will know the best people in your area and may have a working relationship with them. Talk to folks you see in braces. Collect names and opinions. You can also consult the American Association of Orthodontists (AAO) online or by phone. Active members of the AAO are orthodontic specialists. The AAO will give you a list of orthodontists in your area.

Qualifications

Of course, the orthodontist you choose must have all the necessary qualifications. Orthodontists themselves strongly urge you to be sure that the AAO emblem is on display. This ensures that you are being treated by a "Professional who has completed advanced education required by the American Dental Association to permit announcement as 'specialist in orthodontics'" (AAO pamphlet "Facts About Orthodontics).

Chair-Side Manner

Beyond the professional qualifications, be sure that the orthodontist is someone you like because you will see a great deal of him over the years. What style of doctor do you most enjoy or tolerate? How does this practitioner communicate with patients? Ask if there are regular conferences during treatment and ask about access to your doctor when you are not in her office. For instance, one doctor pays a person (who is not an orthodontist) in his office to handle patient communications. She explains treatment, handles questions and deals with the emotional side of the practice while the orthodontist focuses solely on the physical side of the practice.

TIP

A good orthodontist should present you with the following information or make it immediately accessible upon your request before beginning treatment:

•A professional opinion based on looking into your mouth
•A timetable for treatment
•An explanation of the payment schedule and payment options
•Braces-wearing behaviors—dos and don'ts
•Credentials of the orthodontist if they are not in evidence (Does she work primarily with adults?)
•An invitation to get a second opinion

•A description of limitations to your treatment and a reminder that results do not come guaranteed
•A list of potential risks associated with your treatment

Office Style

Check out the atmosphere of the office space. Does it have an open floor plan? Can each patient see and hear each other patient during office visits? If so, will this bother you? Is there a separate waiting room? Where are the sinks where you brush your teeth? Each visit typically starts with brushing. Consider your privacy threshold for all these issues as regards the space you see before you.

Talk to folks in the waiting room. Ask how treatment is progressing and the length of a typical wait. Some very good orthodontists become so popular that they take on too many patients, overbook and keep patients waiting every day. Consider that an overbooked orthodontist may translate into a protracted treatment calendar!

SOUND BITE

One braces wearer, over fifty years old, complains that at his orthodontist's largely pediatric practice the assistants seem unable to change manner when speaking to him. He is irritated and doesn't feel respected when they talk to him as if he is a child.

SOUND BITE

I am frustrated because I think my doctor has way too many patients. I think everyone is in braces for too long. I have to make appointments three or four months in advance.
JoAnn

How far away is that orthodontic office? Remember that you may be visiting there every month to six weeks for the whole treatment time. Consider that commute! The drive and the parking will be forever etched in the authors' memories.

Treatment Choices

If you have decided on treatment, remember that your mouth still belongs to you. This is not to say that treatment is whimsical. Follow your orthodontist's treatment prescription but keep your preferences and opinions clear. If your orthodontist says you will need to have your jaw broken to help your bite, it's o.k. to decline. It is your jaw and you need to decide if the treatment plan works for you. Ask what the consequences may be of a different choice. For example, would the outcome suffer if you left your jaw alone? For major events, such as surgery, it is wise to get a second opinion.

TIP

Clue your doctor in to what else is going on in your life so that he can adjust treatment accordingly.

SOUND BITE

One fellow I met skiing cheerfully proscribed doing whatever the most drastic suggestions were from your orthodontist. His theory: the process went much faster that way. His own treatment had gone quickly and well and had involved breaking his jaw (jaw surgery). He had a great attitude and was completely unruffled by his braces.

Pam

Some less serious but more obvious choices involve the look of your braces. Brackets (see glossary) come in a variety of ceramics, metals, and plastics. Not every orthodontist has each type available. The plastic can be nearly invisible, especially if the loops you choose are clear. However, if you like Indian food, red wine or mustard, your clear loops will stain rendering those "invisible" braces highly and grungily visible. The clear plastic brackets are not worth the extra cost if those are foods you enjoy.

SOUND BITE

I had silver tops and bottoms and wore a lot of silver jewelry.

Jeannie

Perhaps you would like your braces to be entirely

invisible. Invisalign ™ touts itself as an alternative to

wearing bands and brackets.

> Invisalign ™ is a new and exciting
> technology in orthodontics. We use it in
> specific cases on our adult patients with
> great success. It is a cosmetic alternative
> to traditional braces, but it has its
> limitations as to what types of cases it will
> work on. Generally speaking, patients with
> minor crowding or spacing that have a
> good bite can be candidates. Those with
> severe crowding and problems with the
> bite may not be candidates for the
> procedure. You should schedule an
> examination to find out what options are
> available for you and to determine if this
> procedure is right for you.
>
> Randall Markonian and Jeffrey
> Mastroianni, ThinkBraces.com

Neither of the authors were candidates for

treatment like Invisalign ™. Lynn's teeth had to

be moved too far. Pam's teeth were too crowded

and overlapping.

One Invisalign ™ candidate described her surprise that the process was not as invisible as she had wished. While no one could see that she was wearing orthodontia, the orthodontia changed her appearance, and because of its invisibility, did not explain why she had temporary gaps between teeth here and there. She wished the orthodontist had told her of the possibility of these interim changes before she had chosen treatment and ended up opting out part way through.

SOUND BITE

In some interim stages of treatment it is possible to look kind of weird. If you just want to make small adjustments (to the look of your teeth) you may find along the way that things look worse before they look better. But without the explanation of (visible) braces, it just looks strange. And defeats the purpose of Invisalign™.

Margaret

Adult Treatment

Many of us first go to an orthodontist based on a recommendation from our dentists. If you visit an orthodontist for a consultation, likely you will hear of ways in which you can benefit from orthodontia in a message similar to this:

> When left untreated, many orthodontic problems become worse. Treatment by a specialist to correct the problem is often less costly than the additional dental care required to treat the serious problems that can develop in later years.
>
> The importance of an attractive smile should not be underestimated. A pleasing appearance is a vital asset to one's self-confidence. A person's self-esteem often improves as treatment brings teeth, lips and face into harmony. In this way, orthodontic treatment can benefit social and career success as well as improve one's general attitude toward life.
>
> AAO pamphlet "Facts About Orthodontics"

Quite a hefty promise!

SOUND BITE

I had to sit down with my orthodontist [several months into treatment] and tell him that my sense of perfection was different from his. As far as I was concerned my mouth was perfect. For me the treatment was a success and it was time for the braces to come off.
Jenny

Be mindful that, as a group, orthodontists are perfectionists. Decide how much you want perfection for yourself. Regardless of the depth and excellence of their combined expertise, the orthodontists cannot decide for you. You may decide that if it ain't broke, the orthodontist has nothing to fix or that at a certain point has fixed enough.

For those of you now seeking a solution as adults, take heart. According to the AAO a quarter of orthodontic patients are adults. You will have company in the waiting room, at the grocery store, and possibly at work. And if your gums, teeth, and supporting bone are healthy, then orthodontic success is a strong likelihood.

Chapter 2

What is Treatment?

Your treatment is designed specifically for you and your problem. Your orthodontist will make equipment for your mouth alone, with the fundamental idea of exerting pressure to move your teeth into their proper positions. In response to the pressure, your body creates new supporting tissue for the teeth.

Although each person's treatment plan is unique, there are some constants. Below we describe the characteristics of the different kinds of office visits.

Initial Inspection

First the orthodontist will want to examine your mouth and learn your orthodontic and dental history.

Likely he will look at you in profile and facing forward, and also examine your teeth and your bite. For this visit you get to sit in that really comfy, expensive chair.

Planning and Consultation

Many patients then have a second appointment at the orthodontist's desk, and sit in a less comfortable chair, to discuss logistics. Before treatment begins, your orthodontist will likely square away financial matters, discuss the treatment schedule and procedures, and ask for your signature here and there. Some orthodontists request that patients bring their significant others to this meeting. These orthodontists understand the need for those close to the braces-wearer to be informed. Your life is about to change.

Records

Most first treatment visits involve x-rays, photos
and impressions (plaster models) made of one's teeth.
The orthodontist calls this a "records" visit. It is repeated
after the braces come off for comparison and contrast.
Your orthodontist may photograph you from the front and
sides first. He may ask you to move your jaws in different
ways for different photos. Many, many photos.

You might expect to feel self-conscious about
having pictures taken, but you might not expect
discomfort. The challenge for the orthodontist is
gathering detailed data from a small space. Photos of the
interior of the mouth may involve inserting a mirror in
your mouth and holding a pose with the hard, shiny
rectangle propping your lips open—not exactly
comfortable.

TIP

Take prophylactic pain-killers for the records visit.

Routine Treatment Visits

The authors accompanied each other to a routine office visit to compare experiences. Both offices have sign-ins asking time of arrival. One waiting room includes space for children to play. After a short wait, we were each called to the chair for the exam. One practice seated us in privacy; at the other, we were seated in a larger open space with other patients within ear-shot. Patients who want a private consultation can do so behind the doctor's office door.

Our visits proceeded like this: brush teeth, get wire removed, brush and floss with wire off, sit for doctor's exam and wire adjustments, sit for assistant to insert the newly-adjusted wire, schedule new appointments.

TIP

Wear Chap Stick or lip-gloss for your orthodontic appointments. Your lips might get vigorously stretched in all directions during the visit. Chapped lips crack and hurt.

Depending on how often your orthodontist sees you, your office visit may be a brief check-up to be sure the wires are firmly in their brackets, the alastics (see glossary) are all in place, the wire ties are in the right locations, and your gums look good. And you are out the door in fifteen minutes. Other visits require changing wires and affixing them with new alastics, wire ties and/or chains. This type of visit can take an hour or more.

TIP

If your wires are to be changed, request the opportunity to floss *before* the wires are replaced. It is so easy to floss sans wires that you'll think of it as a treat. (Cheap thrills? Maybe, but you'll tell yourself that when the braces finally do come off, flossing will seem such a snap that you'll never miss a day.)

Some orthodontists check the articulation between upper and lower teeth each visit. Their patients become used to the mantra, "Bite down. Again. Bite down. Relax your jaw. Now bite down again. Once more ..." Towards the end of the treatment the orthodontist may use articulating paper, often called occlusal paper. You will be asked to tap your teeth together with the paper slipped in between upper and lower jaws. Your teeth will mark the high areas that then can be ground down to allow for a better bite fit.

Some orthodontists will require that x-ray films be taken in order to visualize the movement of the roots. These films may be taken in the office or in a radiology lab. Expect two or three of these sessions during the span of your treatment.

There may be a need at some point to make a mold of your top teeth in order to have a bite plate made.

This only takes a minute. Another mold will be made at the end of treatment in order to make retainers.

TIP

Given the choice between bubblegum and berry, when getting an impression, choose bubblegum! BUT mint is best, if available.

Lynn

You may need to have teeth removed if your problem is crowding. The orthodontist will include this option only if removing teeth improves your chances of success. Conversely, the orthodontist might have to reduce a space. If you have gaps from missing teeth, the orthodontist may plan for prosthetics to fill them.

The equipment you wear changes over the course of treatment. Initially wires are light-gauge and there may be expanders or springs. An intermediate stage consists of heavier gauge wire without additional contraptions. Just when you may think that everything is getting easy, because your teeth look straight and the springs are gone, a new twist may be added. Elastics! These small rubber bands, positioned from upper to lower jaw, move the jaw into a new position. For instance, in the case of a cross bite. Each visit your doctor will update you on the position in which to wear them and will supply you with a small bag of the tiny elastics. Sometimes these are worn only at night, but you may be required to wear them during the day as well.

TIP

Try hooking the elastics by yourself before you head home so that the orthodontist or the assistant can confirm that you know the proper configuration.

SOUND BITE

Every night for more than a year I had to hook my jaws shut with rubber bands. This put a crimp on my love life but closed my bite substantially.
                                    Pam

Debonding and Retainers

The day has come! Party! But wait ... Getting the braces off takes a little time. Each bracket and band must be plucked off individually. Expect some pressure as the torque required to separate (debond) the tooth from the cement is substantial.

Many orthodontists will scrub your teeth after the hardware is out of the mouth. Others suggest scheduling a cleaning appointment with your dentist soon after the braces come off. Assess your appearance! Smile! Ta-da!

SOUND BITE

My orthodontist presents you with a bottle of sparkling cider and a big balloon.
Lynn

To give your new look its fullest brilliance, you may choose to bleach your teeth. The dentist will happily accommodate, but there are also a variety of over-the-counter kits that are easy and effective.

In one's delight to get the braces removed, it is easy to forget that having the braces off means putting the retainers on. Once the braces are removed, the orthodontist will fit you for a retainer or retainers. Often you must return the following day to pick up a temporary retainer. These are customarily made of a clear, light plastic. Within a couple of weeks the permanent retainer will be ready. This is made from a more substantial plastic and may include a wire embedded or attached.

Retainer Checks

Many orthodontists leave their patients to their own devices once they have been equipped with retainers. Some doctors will ask you to visit annually for a retainer check. At these visits, the doctor makes sure that the retainers are doing their job and that the teeth are remaining stable.

Glossary of Equipment

Alastics or **ligature ties** loop over the brackets to hold the wires in place. The combination of the alastics and the archwire places the pressure on the teeth that causes them to move. Colored alastics provide a fun form of self-expression. Many kids enjoy seasonal colors like black and orange at Halloween, or red, white and blue in July. Black is not only for Goth teenagers. It looks quite sharp. Grey is pretty subtle. Clear alastics are less visible unless they become stained by spices like turmeric and mustard or by red wine. If your wire is removed for each visit then you can choose new colors of alastics each time. If you have the flexible wires, you may be wearing the same color for months. Alastics are part of the basic equipment. They stretch over time and become less effective.

SOUND BITE

Near treatment's end I opted for grey because I was interested in the least noticeable choice. Rainbow is fun. The ugliest combination I got was dark blue and yellow. What possessed me? Fluorescent green alastics got the most noise!
Pam

Archwires (Wires) shove into a groove in the brackets and tie down, or slip into a tube on the bands. The wires allow the use of one tooth as leverage against another. Each time the orthodontist replaces the wires, he may increase the gauge. Wires may pop out easily early in treatment. Be respectful of that "don't" food list that you were given.

There are two main styles of treatment. One involves a flexible wire that pulls fairly steadily the entire time between visits. The other uses a stiffer wire that pulls hard right after the appointment, changing the teeth very rapidly and then stabilizing them until the next appointment. The same wire may be used in your mouth for months in succession with changes made to its shape in order to push or pull different teeth.

Bands affix to the molars. The slots in them and in the brackets hold the wires in place. The bands stay on the teeth throughout treatment.

Bite plates fit against the roof or floor of your mouth. These hard plastic and wire plates protect the palate or the other teeth so that the teeth do not strike against each other. You may be fitted for a bite plate if you have a temporary malocclusion (teeth don't fit together).

Brackets attach to teeth other than molars. These small squares are bonded to each of your front teeth. If you disobey the food rules you can even dislodge one of these. Unless you bust one, you keep these throughout treatment.

Braces may be made of plastic, ceramic or metal. Usually they consist of the brackets, bands, wires, and alastics. The whole contraption.

Chains, like bands, come in a variety of colors. These are like continuous alastics, linking many brackets together. They pull teeth into a straighter line. You may sport these for several months, getting a new one each visit.

Elastics align the bite and close the bite. Remember high school classmates firing these out of their mouths during class? If you have an overbite, under bite, cross bite, or open bite, you may look forward to wearing these. Each bite problem has a different rubber band solution. The elastics come in various gauges depending how much pull is required. Either certain brackets have small hooks or very thin, looped wire hooks are attached to the brackets for use as hooks for the elastics. Elastics often feature in the latter half of treatment. They tend to follow the major straightening of teeth. Some regimens call for wearing one or two elastics around the clock. At other times, you may only have to wear them at night.

Expanders or **Hyrax** enlarge the palate. For adults, this process may involve surgery to cut the bone in the roof of the mouth first. This natural suture may not be completely knit in a child, permitting the process without surgery. Pushing against the back of the teeth, the expander wires are held together by a crank on a rolling bale, and thus can be adjusted to exert sustained pressure. Sounds fun, right?

Goggles are offered by some orthodontists at every visit to dim the effect of lights in the face and to protect eyes from bits and pieces.

Headgear guides the growth of the face and jaws or anchors the teeth during treatment. It includes a strap worn behind the head to hold the mostly-metal contraption in the mouth.

Lingual braces--the celebrities' choice—attach to the back of the teeth and are fairly difficult to detect. They do not work for many problems according to the authors' orthodontists.

Occlusal paper resembles carbon paper. When bitten upon, it records tooth positions. Orthodontists use it to identify surfaces that might interfere with each other and may grind these down slightly.

Photographs of the inside and outside of the mouth are taken before and after treatment from a variety of angles.

The inside shots may necessitate sliding a mirror into your mouth.

Plaster Models and other **molds** are used for before and after records and to take impressions of your teeth in order to customize braces, mouth plates and retainers. A curved metal pan, full of goo, is inserted in your mouth and held for a couple of minutes while you sit as still as possible. For those with small jaws, this can be painful. (Think prophylactic painkillers for this appointment.) It seems that the folks with the franchise on the metal dishes have a one-size-fits-all mentality. The goo sets and then can be filled with plaster, etc.

Retainers help you settle into your new bite and support your muscles and bones as they adjust to the new positions of your teeth. Retainers are usually made of a hard plastic piece that fits against your palate and a wire that curves in front of your teeth. They can feel more

cumbersome than braces. Where does one's tongue fit?

Many notice new lisping or other enunciation difficulties.

Never fear: full-time wear is temporary.

TIP

Remember not to drink hot fluids while wearing your retainers. You can melt a temporary retainer or alter the fit of a permanent one.

Some retainers are permanent wires placed behind

the teeth and attached with brackets, just like braces.

Often, a small wire, called a lingual retainer, is placed

permanently behind the bottom teeth, just in the front of

the mouth, as a supplement to the lower and upper

removable retainers. This area is hard to support with a

conventional retainer.

Probably for the first six weeks to six months out

of braces you will be asked to wear any retainers night

and day. Later you may wear them just during the night. You may be told to wear them for the rest of your life. If you do not, your teeth will likely revert to their pre-braces look. Consider your expenditures carefully. This is a critical time in which to be compliant. The mouth can shift very rapidly. Teeth move throughout one's lifespan. Failure to wear these devices may render all that treatment time obsolete. One of the authors wore braces as an adult because she failed to wear her retainer from childhood and her teeth reverted.

TIP

WEAR YOUR RETAINERS!

Springs come in a couple of types. Open-coil springs push teeth apart, often to create space in which to rotate a tooth. Closed-coil springs maintain a space, once created. Both are strung onto the arch wire like a bead and held in place by wire ties. They can be quite bulky in the mouth.

Some people have difficulty closing their lips when springs are in place. Usually springs are worn for a very brief spell, perhaps a few weeks or months near the beginning of treatment.

Tie wires attach the archwire to the brackets. These thin wires loop around the bracket. They are tightened by twisting and then they are trimmed so that they won't poke. (That's the plan, anyway. You might like to roll a bit of wax to cover those spots and to protect your mouth's soft parts.)

X-rays allow the orthodontist to see the roots of the teeth. Typically the orthodontist requires a full mouth set before treatment begins and may need them at one or two intervals during treatment to be sure that the roots are lining up as nicely as the visible part of the tooth. Occasionally, the doctor will focus on a specific spot and need an additional couple of x-rays to monitor the migrating of the roots into proper position. It's not advised to be going through treatment while pregnant. After treatment the orthodontist will request another set of x-rays to gauge changes and retention.

Getting Information

Ask Questions. As in any health care situation, one needs to be an informed and active participant in the process.

TIP

Jot down any questions you may have as they occur and keep them in your wallet or purse. That way you don't forget to bring it with you to your appointment—unless, that is, you've also forgotten your driver's license.

What are your possible questions? What is this piece of equipment supposed to do? Should you expect discomfort with a new aspect of treatment? Is there an alternate approach to treatment, a plan B or even plan C?

How long is the treatment expected to last? Are there any

possible complications or anticipated difficulties to guard

against?

Of course there are the small but important things

to remember such as asking for more elastics when you

run out, or asking for wax if you can't get to the drug

store.

SOUND BITE

With adults it would be helpful if the orthodontist would explain the process more— give markers or goals. You know, "By the time we get to point x, you will be able to chew again." I don't expect a treatise on orthodontic theory, but I feel that if I were given some benchmarks, I would be more able to anticipate what's going on.

Randee

Your teeth are straight? Your bite is lined up?

You look done? You were told eighteen months?

Twenty-four? Maybe even thirty? As that closing date

approaches, you become more and more eager or even desperate to become braces-free. You begin to ask your orthodontist, "When will they come off?" We say, "Begin," because you will likely ask your orthodontist this question more than once. According to one orthodontist, that is the question he is asked most frequently. Often an equivocal answer means that the orthodontist simply does not know. He is not concealing information nor trying to frustrate the patient. The orthodontist has to see how the teeth are responding to treatment at each visit. Actual timelines may be impossible to provide.

Timing of Treatment

Planning the definitive family photo session next month? Is the college reunion in May? Dating a brand new person right now? Maybe you have an infant and following anyone else's schedule is problematic?

Consider the landmarks in your life. Go into orthodontia knowing that you may have considerable soreness in the beginning. The braces will probably change your self-image; ultimately, we all hope, for the better. But initially, and sometimes throughout treatment, patients feel less attractive. You may not feel like smiling as much. Negative feelings may even take you somewhat by surprise once the braces are on.

Women who are pregnant or considering getting pregnant soon should realize that treatment involves x-rays. For the doctor to get the full picture and not to have to guess at what the roots are doing, x-rays are essential. How urgent is the orthodontia? Could it wait a few months or a year?

TIP

Minor orthodontic problems can wait if a big event is around the corner. Look at your long-range plans before launching into orthodontia.

Several days after I had my braces put on, I had to speak before a large group at a summer institute. I had to speak all day and be on my feet, very visible and audible. The whole time I was popping Advil and trying to get by on mushy food because I was in pain. If I'd delayed the process just one or two weeks, I wouldn't have a story to tell.

Pam

Length of Treatment

Treatment takes time. Most malocclusion patients (non-traumatic cases) visit the orthodontist every 4 to 6 weeks for 18 months to 3 years. Each appointment lasts anywhere from twenty minutes, on a good day, to two hours, when everything goes askew and a special procedure is on the docket. How does this information affect your current schedule? Can you break away from your other adult activities long enough and often enough? Who's watching the kids? Who's watching your job? One friend, on a very tight timetable, now calls ahead to make sure that the office is running on schedule before driving off to her appointments. Once she missed an important meeting because of a delay there and vowed never again. Call first!

SOUND BITE

The time it takes is huge. It's easy to miss appointments and if I had known it would be so long [two years and counting] I wouldn't have done it again.
        Lisa, who also wore braces as a child

SOUND BITE

It's going to take forever.
                Angela

If your orthodontist says she estimates that treatment will take eighteen months and you plan your wedding to take place one week after this time period, don't be surprised if your wedding photos include shots of you with braces. Remember it is an *estimate*. For your part, you can assure that treatment is going smoothly and on schedule by making and keeping all of the appointments. Also, you can avoid situations that may lengthen treatment time by taking excellent care of your teeth and gums. Other than these interventions, your teeth are not under volitional control and they will move at their own pace, thank you very much. For one wearer we spoke to, this meant two years longer than projected. One woman had her sentence reduced by nearly six months. Other factors may come into play. For example, length of orthodontia required before and/or after accompanying jaw surgery may depend on the course of the post-surgical healing process.

One braces wearer swears she heard, "About one year," as the time estimate. But as she sat in the chair sporting her brand new braces, she was surprised to hear the orthodontic assistant say, "All done. That wasn't so bad, was it? Besides, let's see. It says here they'll be off in twenty months." Twenty months is "about two years," not one year. If you're an impatient type or a precise type you may want to discuss time estimates in detail, including contingency estimates that might be necessary because of possible delays.

SOUND BITE

Jenny's treatment time exceeded the estimate. She was about to be married and requested the removal of her braces. The orthodontist would only agree after she signed a statement along the lines of, "I know I'm asking you to take these off before you want to, but I want to. For me, treatment is over." He removed her braces Monday for a Friday wedding. That week she bleached her teeth—not on everyone's pre-wedding to-do list.

SOUND BITE

I hoped to have my braces off before I turned forty because I figured my children, being very young, would forget what I looked like with braces. Now that I've had them on beyond the estimated treatment time, I don't think that either of them remembers me without braces.
                                                          Pam

TIP

To get the most accurate time estimate, ask the orthodontist: How long does the average

**treatment last? How long have others with my
problems spent in their braces? Will you please
write that projected date of removal on the
front of my file? What is the longest span any
of your patients has spent in braces? Also,
write the date down and ask each time you
visit, "Am I on track for that removal date?"**

At home you'll have to spend more time on your

cleaning routine. The whole procedure of brushing,

flossing, mini-brushing (the little under-the wire brush),

mouth washing and gum stimulating can take twenty

minutes.

TIP

**Break up the cleaning time. Brush and floss
right after supper. Do the rest before bed. Do
the gum stimulating stuff while reading or
watching T.V.**

Dental Visits

Your regularly scheduled visits to the dentist for

cleaning will take a tad longer than they used to with all

that hardware to service.

Some orthodontic patients have difficulty keeping their dental hygiene up to snuff because the wrenching on their teeth may make brushing and flossing hurt. Many dentists will suggest a three-month cleaning interval for them. For patients with extreme difficulty maintaining home hygiene, the recommended span is even shorter. Special prescription rinses help tackle emergent gum disease. Also, dentists may offer samples of different brushes and types of floss. They might have that perfect new tool that actually makes one eager to clean.

TIP

Blueness of the gums means trouble. Call your dentist immediately.

Chapter 3

Your Responsibilities during Treatment

Choosing braces means you need to commit to some behaviors as well as to the braces. Failure to follow the orthodontist's rules could mean that she has to alter the treatment plan, or in extreme cases, stop treating you. Suspending treatment can have terrible consequences for your oral health, far worse than whatever you were going through before treatment. Sound onerous? We are not intending to throw guilt your way, however, the following chapter describes what you must do to be a responsible patient and to ensure the best results from orthodontia.

TIP

Consider carefully what is required to make braces work. If you are not willing to follow the cleaning and diet rules or to keep the payment and appointment schedules, the process will not work. Braces are a substantial investment of time, effort, and bucks. If you can't comply with the rules of treatment, don't start!

Orthodontists expect compliance from adult patients—after all we are grown-ups. In the majority of cases, we make the choice to go into the process ourselves. Since we choose this, doesn't this mean that we will engage fully? You already know the answer. Most of us do really try but psychological factors are meddlesome. Time constraints are genuine. Pain is real. Nevertheless compliance is the best chance you have.

Here's the list:

- FOLLOW INSTRUCTIONS

- CARE FOR APPLIANCES

- KEEP TEETH CLEAN

- PAY ON TIME

- MAKE AND KEEP APPOINTMENTS

- COMMUNICATE

- FOLLOW THE BRACES DIET

Follow Instructions

So, the orthodontist says you need a bite plate and his assistant gives you an information sheet exhorting you to keep it in at all times, except when brushing. You go out to dinner with friends and decide to jettison the bite plate in order to eat more heartily. You discreetly wrap the bite plate in your paper napkin. You get home that evening and discover the bite plate is missing but decide you cannot bring yourself to search in the Dumpster out back of the restaurant, opting instead to pay $----.00 to replace your bite plate.

Or, you decide that you've got to have diet cola, because that's what you drink all day at your desk, and you just can't brush while you're at work because there is no time. Later, when your braces are removed you—and everyone else—notice irreversible and unsightly white marks on your front teeth caused by the phosphoric acid in the soda. Your orthodontist is kindly, however, and refrains from saying, "I told you so." Get the point? Follow directions.

Care for Your Teeth and Your Appliances

This is going to take a little time. First of all you should brush after you eat—every time you eat. This is because if you don't regularly get rid of the plaque that builds up around the braces it can cause decalcification around the base of the brackets which can mean permanent, ugly white marks on the surface of your teeth. After all those months of braces do you really want to have to see permanent white outlines around the places where the brackets were cemented? I think not. But the thing that will keep you brushing is the bad breath that haunts the non-brusher. The sticky white stuff that collects on your teeth is called plaque. Bacteria + Food Particles + Saliva = Plaque + Really Bad Breath. So, carry a travel-sized toothbrush with you. Your friends will thank you.

TIP

Put your bite plate in fizzy cleaner (anything made for dentures) while you shower.

SOUND BITE

The hardest thing is not feeling like my teeth are clean—it is a big time commitment to clean these puppies.
                                                Randee

Take stock while flossing. Keep an eye out for wires that may have slipped out of brackets or anything that seems to be poking when it didn't before. As soon as you notice, report problems with equipment. Also report any unusual or continuing soreness or pain in teeth or gums. Usually the orthodontist will want to see you right away.

Accustomed to no more than toothpaste, brush, and floss? Never heard of sulcus brushes? Never knew someone could make a living selling them? Braces may change your vocabulary and your perspective. The big message: keep your mouth clean. When your mouth feels tender after the wires have been tightened, Water Piks ™ and rinses are good solutions. Electric toothbrushes may hurt less than regular brushes. Below we list many of the tools you will need to use.

Glossary of Cleaning and Care Equipment

Denture cleaners aren't just for dentures anymore! These tablets dissolve in water to form a bubbly cleaning concoction for any removable hardware.

Floss options include regular old floss and a **threader**. The threader is a large, flexible, thin plastic needle. Flossing takes time and dexterity, as the floss must be threaded between the gum and the wire. It is rather like sewing. Some folks just straighten the tip of their waxed floss instead and manage to thread that under the wires. You can also use floss which comes in measured lengths with a stiffened end (one brand is Thornton ™) which can easily be threaded between the teeth and wires, thus eliminating the need for a threader.

Fluoride Gel can be put on the gums and left on overnight. This encourages healthy gums.

Paste is paste. Nothing special here, except to avoid whitening tooth pastes since they will leave you with a spotty look when the braces come off.

Retainer washes resemble denture cleaners. The retainers sit in a frothy bath for at least 15 minutes a day to remove tartar build up.

Toothbrushes come in an amazing number of styles:

Baby toothbrushes fit between the brackets and the gum line. Buy one of these and use it a couple of times a week in addition to your routine to be sure the gums are adequately stimulated.

Cylindrical brushes are the best! These tiny brushes fit between the wires and the teeth. They can be inserted from the top or the bottom of the wire. These clean where all other brushes cannot reach.

Electric toothbrushes are easy and hurt less than a conventional brush.

SOUND BITE

After I started using an electric brush, my dentist switched me from three- to four- month cleaning intervals. When I first got my braces my mouth was so sore that regular brushing hurt. I developed gingivitis because I skimped on brushing, waiting for the pain to subside. As soon as I bought an electric brush my hygiene improved. My dentist says that electric brushes and braces are made for each other.

Pam

Orthodontic brushes have a long furrow down the middle designed to fit around the braces, so that the brush can reach the tooth above and below the brackets.

Regular toothbrushes have their limitations. They do not fit in many of the new and interesting crevices that appear once one is braced. You might find that using a brush with a small, soft head is best.

Sulcus brushes look a bit like the toothbrush assembly line ran out of bristle. They have a bit of bristle just at the head end. This small head is designed to be rubbed along the gum or sulcus line to ward off gingivitis.

Toothpicks get mixed responses from dentists and orthodontists. Metal toothpicks and scrapers are available at many large pharmacies even though the dentists and orthodontists will probably caution you against using these at home. They can scratch the enamel. Wooden toothpicks are frequently recommended. Rubber toothpicks are great gum stimulants.

Washes reach where floss and brushes may not penetrate. This is particularly important if you have gingivitis. A very strong antibacterial prescription wash helps prevent gum disease when brushing is painful. Without healthy gums, you might as well give up on the whole shebang.

Water Piks ™ wash food particles from hard to reach spots with a jet of water. The water tank may also be filled with fluoride rinses.

Wax protects the inside of your mouth from poking wires and sharp protrusions of the brackets. Rip a piece from the thin rods. Roll it into a ball and press it gently onto the offending hardware. It can bring instant relief. Unfortunately, chewing is probably the most painful thing to do with bristly hardware and wax usually won't stay on while eating. You may choose whether to remove it before you eat, in the privacy of the bathroom, or just swallow it, as it won't harm you. Last time you ate wax was crayons in preschool …

SOUND BITE

Two years into his treatment, Daren smiled broadly as he described socializing during the early days. Smiling hurt at the beginning and going out for a beer with his friends and laughing over their jokes made his mouth sore. He remembers that wax saved him.

Keep Teeth Clean on the Road

Whether you are away from home just for the day or on long trips, bring: dental floss, toothbrush, toothpaste, wax, a small brush for between teeth and braces and a mirror (or note where a mirror is handy upon entering a room). While traveling it never seems to fail that that a wire, innocently unnoticeable before departure, suddenly starts to poke. Don't be hoodwinked. You may not have used wax for months, but do not leave it at home!

SOUND BITE

I also carry a small metal travel toothpick and mouthwash. If this sounds like too much gear, remember you can get travel sized toothpaste, mouthwash, a travel toothbrush and small round versions of packaged dental floss. If a mishap occurs, say a broken bracket or wire, wearers report that they have had little trouble finding a local orthodontist to evaluate the situation, though she may only be able or willing to provide a temporary solution. One braces wearer reports having had to use nail clippers to extricate herself from a jabbing bit of broken wire.

Lynn

Pay Bills

Don't forget to keep to your payment schedule if not to honor your obligation, then to appease the orthodontist. After all she is standing over you with pliers and snippers and other sharp instruments.

SOUND BITE

Dad worked hard to pay for it the first time. (This second time) It was free [yeah, "free"] because of the insurance.

Lisa

The cost of treatment will vary depending on the extent and severity of your particular problem. However even at the low end you can assume that treatment *ain't cheap*. One way of looking at it is that the money spent now on orthodontia can ultimately save you money on future dental bills to treat more serious problems. It can save your teeth so that when you're eighty, you're not wearing dentures. The cost in additional dental care needed because of malocclusion problems can actually exceed that for orthodontic treatment. One dentist compared it to painting your house when the paint shows slight signs of peeling rather than waiting until the raw wood has been exposed to the weather so long that it develops dry rot and the wood siding has to be replaced. If you have a dental plan it may include orthodontic benefits, if only partial coverage. Also most orthodontists will discuss treatment options and prices with you and can arrange a monthly payment schedule, usually after an initial down payment. While it would be imprudent to quote the price of orthodontia given all the variables, suffice it to say that the cost is more than that of a refrigerator and less than the cost of a car.

SOUND BITE

A woman reported discussing the cost of orthodontia with her mother at lunch one day. The mother felt badly that she hadn't been able to afford orthodontia when her daughter was young and she wrote out a check for the entire treatment, saying she couldn't afford it then, but she could and would now.

Make and Keep Appointments

This is in your own best interest. The progression from one stage to the next can't happen if you regularly show up two or three weeks after a scheduled appointment. You can shave off weeks or even months of your treatment if you keep every appointment. If you need appointments at particular times of the day, the receptionist might not want to oblige you if you've blown appointments with no-shows. Not many orthodontists work evenings and weekends, so the early-in-the-day and late-in-the-day appointments are hot properties.

Communicate

It is important to communicate to your orthodontist any changes that you notice. If a tooth or jaw is aching, this information helps him in determining how to adjust the braces. Often the patient can *feel* what the orthodontist has a hard time seeing. A broken bit of tooth or a loose crown can cause problems if left untended. Unlike your orthodontist or dentist, you see and feel your mouth daily and have the most recent information on its progress. Never assume that your mouth is behaving like everyone else's and that the orthodontist has seen every situation a million times and can tell without your feedback exactly what is occurring in your mouth. Say, "This wire pokes me." "This chafes." "My lips stick out so I can't close my mouth all the way."

"I'm snoring and bugging my spouse. I never used to."

"My teeth hurt for four days after tightening." You get the picture.

Follow the Braces Diet

Know those eating rules before you get braced. If you are unwilling or unable to follow the rules, treatment will likely fail.

SOUND BITE

Polly wore braces for one weekend before insisting on their removal. She learned after the brackets had been bonded that she wouldn't be able to eat her favorite snack, Power Bars ™ (about 50% of her caloric intake some days). The lifestyle change was too dramatic. She chose prosthetics instead.

Chapter 4

Pain, Problems, and Changes

Pain

There's pain in the chair, pain in the aftermath of an appointment, and pain from daily wear. Ok, pain is subjective. In our interviews we found a range of responses to the discomfort. For some it seemed barely noticeable. For others it was a daily aggravation.

Pain in the chair may result from sharp tools including x-ray film, pressure on sore teeth, overstretching of lips, and tired jaw from keeping it open.

SOUND BITE

Before appointments I take two Ibuprofen and then a couple every four hours. The pain never goes away completely, but it is dulled to a tolerable level. The key really is just to stay busy.
Randee

SOUND BITE

A lot of people told me that the worst was after getting the wire tightened. I think the worst is the week before the appointment. All the wires are sticking out.

Dan

TIP

Let your orthodontist know if your pain threshold is low. (You are not a wimp!)

SOUND BITE/TIP

Occasionally during your visits the assistant may have to put some pressure on a tooth. My favorite assistant always warns me and has me press with my finger or tongue on the other side of the tooth to equalize the pressure. I also use the most powerful tool ever taught me: breathing. Breathing got me through two labors without drugs. Make your breath slow and deep and it will help.

Pam

The discomfort inherent in having all of those wires and brackets inside of one's mouth varies from individual to individual. Some experience inflammation and discomfort on the inside of the mouth for only a couple of weeks after braces are placed. Others seem to have semi-uncomfortable mouth during the whole course of treatment. Still others have only intermittent soreness for which the application of dental wax, to smooth the surfaces of the wires and brackets, seems to do the trick.

Jaw pain can happen at any point. Sometimes it is the result of malocclusion and the resultant effort of chewing on mismatched surfaces. Other times jaw pain occurs because of grinding or clenching the jaw, either consciously, to confirm the temporary but irritating feeling of one's molars not coming together, or unconsciously. At any rate, any anti-inflammatory/analgesic will usually be sufficient to take the edge off. One braces wearer had as her standard, *"Tylenol before and a beer after."*

TIP

Always have wax on hand.

Problems associated with Treatment

Accidents

Happenstance accounts for a small percentage of complications with braces—car, bike, and skiing accidents, any blow to the mouth that can displace either braces or teeth. If you get whacked in the face when you are in braces, you can be more severely injured than you would have been without them.

> ### *SOUND BITE*
>
> ***But, sometimes, the braces are what save you: One young patient was riding her bike with her dog on a leash. Her dog went one way around a pole; she went the other. Her face went into the pole. The braces were a godsend. She did have a few extra months of treatment but all her teeth were saved.***

Adult Mouths

Complications with braces are more likely for adults than for children. Our faces have stopped growing. From the outset wearing braces as adults is a compromise. A variety of small and large-scale problems can crop up—we can lose teeth, our gums may break down, or we may develop temporomandibular joint disorder. Your orthodontist cannot guarantee that you will be able to avoid these problems. Such complications make adult care a cooperative venture with other types of doctors, including radiologists, periodontists, endodontists, dentists, orthognathic surgeons, plastic surgeons, prosthodontists, pathologists, and restorative surgeons.

SOUND BITE

The teeth on my left side didn't meet after my second surgery. My mouth was wired shut, so there was nothing that my orthodontist could do [to advance treatment until the wires were removed].

JoAnn

Ankylosed tooth

An infrequent event is an ankylosed tooth, one so firmly attached to the jawbone that it will not move. That tooth can be extracted or, in some cases, surgically moved.

Bonding and Debonding

Putting on and taking off the braces will occasionally damage a tooth, especially if it had cracks or cavities before. It is sobering to think that after more than four years in braces such a catastrophe could occur.

Broken Dietary Rules

Things may go south because of failure to adhere to dietary restrictions. Popcorn husks wedged between braces and gums can cause inflammation. Swiping one of your son's Now and Laters™ (hard, chewy taffy) can pop off a bracket or bend a wire. When tempted to eat forbidden foods, think: a minute in the mouth, an hour in the chair—plus travel time.

Discoloration

A tooth that has had a bad history may discolor when the braces are on, calling for a root canal. After treatment, bleaching may solve this.

Headgear, etc.

The extra equipment you might be asked to wear could hurt you. Remove headgear and neck gear only after easing the tension on the unit. Snapping at the gear can injure the face or eyes. And you are never supposed to wear headgear while engaged in sports. Would you want to?

Moving

If you move in the middle of treatment, you may find it hard to locate an orthodontist who will proceed exactly as your prior doctor did. Each doctor has his own style and some orthodontists may be uncomfortable taking on someone else's patient. They may differ in approach. Insurance coverage may also differ and suddenly land you with a larger financial burden. For example, there may be a big fee levied before taking off the braces.

SOUND BITE

In the midst of treatment, Julianne decided to take her braces off prematurely rather than wear them in the same configuration for six months. She was heading off on an extended stay overseas and did not want to investigate the realm of foreign orthodontics.

TIP

Before moving, get a list of recommendations from your current doctor. Phone these people ahead of time. Explain your move and name your doctor as the "recommender." This way your potential doctor will be able to determine if you are a match for his style of practice.

Orthodontic treatment varies dramatically from country to country. In some places it is unavailable. The United States and Canada set high standards for the practice. In these countries straight teeth are the societal norm. This is not true of most of our planet.

Periodontal Disease

If, in the course of treatment, you find that your gums swell or change color, it is imperative that you contact your dentist. If your mouth is too sore to clean effectively, she can give you special rinses and schedule more frequent professional cleanings. When periodontal disease runs unchecked, it can lead to receding gums, loss of supportive bone for the teeth, and loss of the teeth themselves. A periodontist may be called in to help control the problems. If they are not stoppable, the braces may have to be removed.

Poor Hygiene

The most common reason for the failure of orthodontia reported by our orthodontists is lack of

patient cooperation, meaning poor hygiene. Gums do not fare well when bacteria lounge about too long. Adults overlook flossing and brushing because we are less concrete-operational than kids and can rationalize that we will do it first thing, (pick one): tomorrow morning, when we get to work, when we get home, etc. Be vigilant about the health of your mouth. Otherwise, you may be choosing cavities, periodontal disease, staining, and decalcification of your teeth.

Braces do not produce stains and cavities; people do.

Relapse

Another sobering thought is the risk of relapse. Relapse means that your teeth and jaw regress to their pretreatment positions. Do not believe that your teeth are locked into place because you are an adult. Teeth can move any time. The lower front teeth move especially easily. Various behaviors contribute to relapse including not wearing your retainer as the doctor instructed, mouth breathing, tongue thrusting, immature swallowing (the tongue pushes against the front lowers), and periodontal disease. Magical as your orthodontist may be, he cannot guarantee against all of these. Your best bet, if you choose to wear braces, is to see the process as life-long, including maintenance after the Braces–Are–Off Party.

Root Resorption

Roots may shorten during treatment. If the root gets too short, the patient could lose a tooth. This can occur if teeth move too rapidly, causing the roots to shear off due to the pressure (called *root shear*). Wearing braces longer may also increase the odds of developing this condition; however, a little bit of root change is not supposed to be dangerous. No one knows who is predisposed. Your dentist and orthodontist should work together to monitor this situation by visual inspection and x-rays.

Swallowing and Inhaling Parts

Yikes. There is a small risk. Either during an appointment when bits are loose, or outside of the office, particularly if you have engaged in eating the crunchy or sticky prohibited foods, it is possible to dislodge or to break off pieces of your braces and to swallow them. This has never happened to anybody to whom we spoke.

Temporary Malocclusion and Grinding

Teeth move around. These constant shifts may cause them to bump or grind against each other in ways that hurt or are potentially damaging to the teeth. Enamel can be lost. Controlling these "meetings" is very tricky for the orthodontist because of the constant state of flux.

A specialist might have to make you a bite plate to separate the occlusal surfaces.

Sometimes the braces themselves are the source of the difficulty. If you grind your teeth and have chosen ceramic braces, you may worsen the wear to your teeth as they come in contact with the braces. Your orthodontist may recommend against ceramics if you are a known grinder.

Temporomandibular Joint Disorder (TMJ)

TMJ symptoms have not been conclusively linked to bad bites. If you experience significant jaw-joint pain, it is unlikely that braces will make it go away. TMJ may mean you will not be able to wear elastics as part of your treatment. You might have to rely on a TMJ specialist.

Other Specialists

In addition to the regular visits with your orthodontist, dentist, and radiologist, visits with other specialists might become part of your treatment. The list below includes the types of doctors most commonly involved in associated treatments.

Endodontists perform root canal and otherwise care for the pulp of the tooth.

Orthognathic surgeons break jaws—bring the jaw forward or back if elastics and bite plates don't, so as to correct under bites and overbites.

SOUND BITE

Until Daren talked to the third doctor, he didn't believe the message the first had given him, "We're going to have to break your jaw." Thinking the first doctor a quack, Daren put off orthodontia for a couple of years, until he heard the message again and again.

Pathologists treat tumors or lesions. During tooth extractions a different specialist may notice the bump or lesion and refer you for a biopsy.

Periodontists specialize in gums. They perform gum grafts in the case of recession and may remove gum tissue around a misaligned tooth. Periodontal problems may lead to orthodontic ones and vice versa.

Plastic surgeons address trauma to soft tissue (perhaps after an accident) and may recommend that you stabilize teeth with braces after their treatment.

Prosthodontists make false teeth and work with patients who have suffered a major trauma. For example, a person may be missing part of the jaw because of a cancer. The prosthodontist works in concert with the restorative oral surgeon or the dentist to customize missing sections of the jaw.

Restorative dentists build crowns and bridges, implants and build-ups if a tooth is broken, missing, or chipped. Orthodontists will refer for implants whenever cuts to the tissue or bone are required.

Temporomandibular disorder specialists may be physical therapists or stress-control specialists who help treat temporomandibular (jaw) joint disorders such as chronic earache and headache.

The fine print: associated with all medical procedures is risk of complication. Discuss the likelihood and details with any specialist you might see in addition to your orthodontist.

SOUND BITE

My doctor told me I should cover all the mirrors in the house; I'll look like a pumpkin.
Dan, before orthognathic surgery

TIP

If at all possible when you get surgery, stay home for the maximum time recommended instead of going straight back to work.

Physical and Emotional Changes

SOUND BITE

I had a lot of men talk to me. It's such a conversation piece. People are intrigued that an old coot would have these braces.
Jeannie

SOUND BITE

I didn't think that it affected how I looked that much.
Gilles

Most of the physical changes resulting from braces are small-scale but not necessarily subtle. Of course, the biggest change will be the appearance and feel of your face, particularly your mouth. Reshaping the teeth alters the soft tissue above. Faces can begin to look different, especially to their owners. Other than you, dentists and family members will be the most likely candidates to recognize the changes. One dentist announced to a braced-one, "Now you have a chin!"

Expectations and Adjusting to Life after Braces

Are you expecting a picture-perfect smile? Less self-consciousness about crooked teeth? Easier cleaning? A more comfortable bite? Most braces wearers report outcomes that meet or exceed their expectations.

If your previous poor bite was contributing to temporomandibular joint pain, you may find that this problem has gone away after braces. Life is happier without pain. You will be smiling more.

If your pre-braces condition was cosmetically displeasing, you will rejoice at having straight teeth. For most folks the change vastly enhances a person's looks. (Remember that while orthodontia may modify the configuration of your teeth, it will not give you *new* teeth. They will still be the same old tusks unless you decide on surfacing or caps.)

With a better bite most people also gain better oral health—important if you want your own teeth when you're old. Flossing is a snap and you have fewer places for stringy foods or seeds to get stuck. The whole cleaning process is abbreviated. Halleluiah!

Less obvious benefits of a better bite? An improved ability to chomp into a whole apple and to snip off the stray thread on your sleeve with your front incisors!

While most of these changes after braces sound great and are, some find it difficult to adjust to them nevertheless. For instance one former braces wearer found it impossible to nibble her cuticles with any accuracy, a habit that had given her four decades of solace in anxiety-producing situations.

Some people report that it took time to get used to a different way of chewing, especially because they had dealt with poor occlusion for years and had developed funny patterns.

Your speech might change subtly or not so subtly.

For a very small number, the braces produced minor problems—with simple fixes. Two people mentioned having unstable incisors after the braces were removed necessitating a permanent retainer cemented behind the front teeth.

Straightened teeth can change the shape of the mouth and hence your overall face shape may be somewhat different. One woman felt her teeth were now so perfect, "I look like I have dentures." Another, with a newly prominent post-braces mouth felt she didn't "look like me." Still another person mourned the loss of the distinctive space between his two front teeth that, in retrospect, had provided him with a distinguishing characteristic he hadn't realized had been so much a part of his self-identity. Most people adjust rapidly and are

thrilled with their new appearance.

Face and Mouth

You may notice that the routine matters of

chewing and talking command your attention because of

the new materials in your mouth and the new shapes

being created there. During treatment some of the

physical changes may not be all together welcome. Many

folks notice slight lisps and similar minor awkwardness

in their speech because it's hard to navigate around all the

stuff in the mouth. New spaces may open and shut,

altering how breath travels through the mouth. Some letters can suddenly sound windy.

The way one's mouth feels is also different. How one's lips move to cover the teeth, where the tongue presses to make certain sounds, how one breathes at night—when elastics are closing a usually open mouth, for example—all of these will be transformed. For some of us, this adjustment is arduous, for others, mundane.

SOUND BITE

It wasn't particularly difficult. It was a minor scenario. I didn't have any surgery or anything.
Gilles

A few treatment procedures involve short-term stints in which teeth are pushed apart before they are pulled into line. During the pushing phase, teeth may actually protrude and give a bit of a monkey look. To a lesser extent, a heavily waxed wire can create this look too. These phases can make one feel unattractive and can bring about serious doubts as to the wisdom of the braces idea. Some people retreat and spend as much time as possible at home; they are so self-conscious. Some stop dating and attending parties. Try to remember that the changes are short-lived, that you really do notice the transformation much more than those around you. And remember, too, that your physical appearance is always improved by self-confidence.

Lifestyle

The American Association of Orthodontists is eager to tell you that braces will not interfere with your lifestyle. For example, they say that braces do not prevent one from playing a musical instrument or from singing. However, the braces can create physical changes in the mouth that do prevent certain activities or render them awkward or unfamiliar. The ordinary person can sing or play an instrument but performers may be unable to wear

braces.

SOUND BITE

**The most troublesome part is not being able to
enunciate clearly. When I leave a phone
message, for example, I have to slow way down
and concentrate on speaking clearly.**
                                        Randee

TIP

**Clue your doctor into whatever else is going on
in your life so that he can consider your
priorities during treatment.**

SOUND BITE

**I can't take voice lessons with the braces on
because I can't enunciate clearly enough and
close my mouth all the way.**
                                        JoAnn

Penultimate Chapter

One hard part is that everything looks pretty good

towards the end of braces treatment, perhaps even for a

year or more. You may have weathered your time and wish to return to wireless smiles, easy flossing, and popcorn at movies. The end can be psychologically tough because you must maintain compliance until your treatment is complete. The orthodontist may be waiting until some roots have moved apart or until a bite has closed or until another of a myriad of small instabilities has settled. Remember that the time span told you at the outset of treatment was an approximation. You will be free pretty soon. The more compliant you are, the quicker things will go. We promise.

Self-esteem

The psychological and the physical connect closely. Whether your psyche is giving you mixed, positive, or negative messages may depend on what you *think* you see in the mirror. Braces can feel obvious to the wearer but are unlikely to make much of a stir with friends and workmates.

Braces may make you feel vulnerable. Everyone can see that you need a device to correct a problem. Your appearance has taken a reminiscently adolescent turn. This may feel regressive. But all the while, you know that you are headed toward a brighter smile. That may be enough to sustain you. Your friends and associates may be saying to themselves that you were courageous in your choice to brace yourself and actually be admiring you privately or publicly.

SOUND BITE

Wearing braces gives a younger appearance. I wish I had done it sooner. I'm ashamed I didn't. If you could possibly financially afford it, you should go for it at any age.
>   *Jeannie, out of her braces*

SOUND BITE

I've come a long way in two years.
>   *Danisha*

SOUND BITE

It was something of an imposition, but since it was entirely on the lower jaw, it wasn't evident.
Gilles, out of his braces

SOUND BITE

I think I look better. I'm happy I'm doing it. We're doing a house remodel. This is a piece of cake.
Angela

Self-image may fluctuate throughout treatment.

SOUND BITE

I have to go to meetings with people I just started working with. My bite plate fell off on my tongue. I'm never going to talk again in a group. That kind of thing is very demoralizing.
Lynn

SOUND BITE

I'm ready to get the pliers and pull them off myself.
Pam

SOUND BITE

That's never been a big thing. I'm on the inside.
                    JoAnn

SOUND BITE

I didn't tell anyone [family] in England until
they showed up.

                    Angela

SOUND BITE

It hasn't changed anything drastically. It's O.K.
as an adult to get braces. There is nothing wrong
with it. I'm not upset. I could go either way. I
just want it to be over with.

                    Lisa

SOUND BITE

I'm just a set of teeth.
    Jenny's take on how her orthodontist sees her

Sex

None of those who worried how braces might

affect their sex lives seem to have experienced much

inconvenience—with the exception of holding off on

lengthy bouts of kissing just after the initial placement
and perhaps for a day or two after an adjustment. Of
course, intense brushing is indicated if the relationship is
new and hasn't stood the test of time. One married
woman wore elastics for many months. Every night these
trapped her jaw shut. She felt she had to relinquish many
aspects of her sex life in order to comply with treatment.
One young woman confessed to dating very little and
feeling that she couldn't start any kind of serious
relationship while she was in her braces. She felt less
sexy in them and thought of them as a turn-off.

SOUND BITE

I don't want to kiss. My boyfriend made fun of
me initially.
                                                Lisa

SOUND BITE

You should write a chapter for partners and
spouses! People with braces are
unapproachable: metal mouths. They're
dangerous to kiss. Things are sticking out

everywhere. And you have to listen to the
whining and complaining. For years! I know
it'll be better at the other end, but now we're
waiting for the jaw surgery, both jaws, $20,000.

John, who's partner has been braced for
two years

SOUND BITE

My husband keeps saying, "Why did you do
that?" So much for support! My self-esteem has
plummeted.

Lynn

Smiling

As for smiling—the awkward lips-forced-together

smile of the self-conscious adolescent with braces

needn't be your model. Some braced ones reported

feeling self-conscious during the first few days or weeks,

but the general consensus is that if you naturally smile

with your teeth showing, don't stop now. An unnatural

smile draws more attention to the braces. Friends of

braces wearers say that in little or no time the braces

disappear into the background in the same way eye

glasses tend to become invisible or taken for granted on a

familiar face.

SOUND BITE

I am reluctant to be in pictures, or I won't smile.
I don't like to smile. I worry that there is food in
my teeth.
Lisa

SOUND BITE

As long as I've kept hygienically clean, I don't
really care. I did get plastic ones [braces]
because I want them to be less visible.
JoAnn

SOUND BITE

That's dad's new way of smiling.
Rachel of her braces-wearing father's
lips-together style

Support

Most friends will be supportive. In fact, the

comment most often heard from friends is that they don't

even notice you are wearing braces. We found this hard to believe. What friends probably mean is, "We like you even with your braces," which is indeed a supportive statement. Sometimes a friend or relative will persist in dishing out metal-mouth jokes. Some of these can be funny and are probably meant to cheer you up. One person said she collected all of these jokes and read them over on days when the wires had been adjusted. Sometimes the sympathy makes you want to pull your hair out, like when every person you meet asks when the braces are coming off.

Trauma

Those undergoing orthodontia because of having sustained traumas will encounter more serious and more noticeable physical change. A new jaw may be constructed. A jaw may be wired shut for many months. A plastic surgeon may reconstruct a face. With these enormous challenges, support of family and friends is essential. The orthodontist will likely recommend a professional listener: a counselor, psychiatrist, or psychologist.

Weight

Some braces wearers do lose a few pounds as a result of sore-mouthed-food-avoidance; some, from eliminating certain foods. This weight loss is seldom significant or long-lasting. Even our friend who had her jaw wired shut and ate through a straw for months experienced virtually no weight change. By the way, a chocolate shake rolls in at around 560 calories, over a quarter of a typical daily allotment.

Chapter 5

Surviving Eating

Eating Changes

Once you took eating for granted. You did it frequently and often to excess. You considered it a pleasure and a comfort. While wearing braces you will need to pare, cook, blend or simply avoid.

People with braces face these eating problems: food getting stuck in the braces, dealing with fragile equipment, and soreness in the mouth.

Wires are thin and fragile at the outset. This is a bad time to ignore the rules. Ignoring a rule may bend or pop out your archwires or even snap off a bracket. During the first months of braces you may develop the eating habits of a toddler, breaking off food into little pieces when biting and tearing become difficult. Whole bagels are out. Crunchy carrots are out. Almonds are out. Banana smoothies are in. So is losing a few pounds.

SOUND BITE

From the time the braces are first put in place, your teeth are moving. This means that the occlusal surfaces are probably not going to meet in a comfortable fashion for some time. At times during the treatment I found I could grind on only one molar surface so that most of my chewing was more just rolling the food around, much as my great-grandmother used to gum her food, preferring that to ill-fitting dentures. I found this to be very unsatisfactory both from the point of view of efficiency as well as esthetics. Other people I've spoken with do not remember this as a problem. The way to deal with it? Lower your gustatory expectations; expect to eat for functional purposes rather than for pleasure.

Lynn

SOUND BITE

"You look different."
"Yeah, I know: It's the braces." This was when I had springs in my mouth and looked like Monkey Girl.
"You look thinner."
"Yeah, I know. It's the braces."

I remember this scintillating conversation verbatim because I had it repeatedly. It did not last—the weight loss. I figured out what food was edible.

Pam

SOUND BITE

Everything's been fine. It's just a little hard after they get tightened.

Danisha

TIP

Take the orthodontist's list of prohibited foods seriously. Remember: No popcorn, no hard or chewy candy (nut brittle or taffy) and no gum. And stay away from the destructive and staining effects of soda pop.

SOUND BITE

I didn't eat meat anyway. I kept away from spinach but I didn't really change any habits. I didn't lose a damn pound.

Jeannie

Your mouth can be pretty sore after a visit

especially if the wire has been tightened. However the

soreness may not set in for a few hours and may hurt a

day or two after the visit. We recommend eating something substantial just before the visit in preparation for the softer foods you will be eating when your mouth becomes sore.

Early on, discomfort after an archwire visit may last as long as five days, usually less. Two years into the process, the soreness may only last a day or two and require a couple of soft meals and no Advil™. Some people we interviewed reported that they experienced little or no discomfort at all. We marvel at this.

TIP

Take an Advil™ before your orthodontic visits.

In addition to the soreness issue, there are others. There is the stuff-gets-stuck in the braces issue. This one is mostly esthetic and therefore becomes a matter of importance to your dining companions.

SOUND BITE

With my bridge-thing, I couldn't eat salads and spaghetti.
                                        Lisa

SOUND BITE

The springs seemed to be a magnet for small food particles.
                                        Lynn

If your mouth is wired shut, look into the health food store for the nutritional powders that can be added to drinks. Wheat germ, brewer's yeast and diet powders have good representation in the daily-recommended allowances columns. Many foods can go in the blender and retain flavor but, alas, they do not retain their texture.

TIP

Add salmon to blended soups such as potato.
                        JoAnn

With all of the food restrictions and cautions, what can you eat? Here are some of our soft food favorites. We've also listed foods to avoid simply

because they are too difficult to bite and/or chew.

TIP

Ask other braces wearers about their favorite soft foods. So many resources on-line! You'll find several cookbooks.

Breakfast

TRY

- Yogurt
- Rice pudding (It's not cold like ice cream. A real treat.)
- Cottage cheese
- Hot cereals like oatmeal and Wheateana™
- Blended fruits
- Smoothies
- Custards
- Bananas
- Scrambled eggs

AVOID

- Granola
- Cereals with nuts and dried fruit (hard and chewy!)

- Toast, Bagels, and English muffins unless ripped into little pieces
- Breakfast sandwiches— meats are tough to bite off

<u>The Breakfast Shake</u>

Pam's favorite. It is nutritionally complete for those of you who must drink your meals for an extended period.

1 banana
2 tbsp.—or to taste—frozen orange juice concentrate
¾ c. plain yogurt
¼ c. wheat germ

Blend until smooth. Variations—add other fruits as desired. Also great if you add ice before blending.

Lunch

SOUND BITE

Lunch is not a necessary social occasion any more.

> ***A dentist in braces to her periodontist friend in response to a lunch invitation***

One of the hardest things is being faced with a big bagel sandwich. You're starving and you haven't yet had the experience that tells you this is more than you can handle with sore teeth and braces. Although bagels may not be on most orthodontists' no lists, they are too big and chewy for comfort. Very soft breads are easy to bite but get stuck in the braces.

TRY

- The breakfast list
- Soup
- Pasta
- Mac and cheese
- Tamales
- Casseroles, blends with rice, tofu, well-cooked beans
- Bite-sized foods that you eat with a spoon or fork (that you can carry past your braces)
- Steamed veggies
- Spinach dip
- Risotto

AVOID

- Bagel sandwiches
- Sandwiches on crunchy breads

- Crudités
- Foods that you can't easily break into small pieces (because you will probably have a hard time ripping off pieces with your teeth)

Supper

TRY

- The lunch and breakfast lists
- Boston Market™—or similar delicatessen dishes (BM's chicken is tender enough even right after an archwire session)
- Mashed potatoes
- Squash
- Pumpkin pie
- Indian food—lots of curries are soft, murg bahar, paneer, nan
- Thai food—phad thai, mazuman curries (watch out for the peanuts and staining from turmeric)
- Mexican food—tamales, quesadillas, burritos, (no hard tacos)
- Italian food—pasta is your friend
- Cooked veggies
- Ethiopian food—many soft dishes, very flavorful stews, but full of staining turmeric

Restaurant Dining

Many foods that you may not choose to eat at a business lunch can be eaten any time in the privacy of your own home or in the company of your kind friends. In a restaurant, salads are dangerous; particularly the really good ones with purple and dark green leaves. These are easily trapped in the braces, especially if you have wire ties, elastics, hooks, or chains. Stay away from dark and granular foods as they show up easily when trapped. Soft breads stick and are really ugly. Poppy seeds are a no-go. We recommend choosing something that is easy to fork up and take past your braces.

Avoid appetizers at cocktail parties; many are too big to be popped in the mouth in one mouthful and some are too tough to tear into pieces. Shrimp and stuffed mushrooms come to mind.

Be brave with questions for the wait staff. Ask about preparation details and for recommendations of soft dishes. Some restaurants will gladly substitute mashed potatoes for frites. If your mouth is sore, you may want to order the soup du jour to be brought with everyone else's entrees.

TIP

Eat before or after a business lunch (i.e. in your office with the door closed or in your car).

Sometimes you know that you have food caught in your appliances. Resist the desire to wrestle it free with your finger or your tongue. A swish of water as you're drinking may do the trick. Before dessert run to the WC to do a mirror check. When eating out, absolutely pack floss, toothbrush, mirror, and toothpicks. Our spouses became accustomed to us asking them if we needed to brush. Get someone you trust to signal you if you have anything stuck.

TIP

Try not to have a mealtime job interview.

<u>**AVOID**</u>

- Salads (Those dark leaves can make one look like a chew addict.)
- Spicy food—some of these have ingredients in them that will stain the clear plastic braces (e.g. turmeric, curry, some barbecue sauces and hot sauces)
- Meat—eating meat can mean stringy bits caught between teeth until you are able to floss. It helps if you cut the meat into tiny pieces first.
- Olives (Dark stuff shows on your teeth; what more can we say?)
- Pine nuts (You shouldn't be eating nuts anyway, remember?)
- Soft breads (Very ugly in the braces. These stick readily.)
- Hamburgers (Because of the soft bread.)
- Hard-crust bread (Can break your appliances in the middle of a big event. Oops!)
- Rice (Grains sit very happily above the archwire looking really obvious.)
- Strawberries (Get caught and are highly visible.)
- Shrimp (They're tougher than you think.)
- Stringy veggies (Like sprouts and celery.)
- Poppy seeds
- Raisins
- Corn chips (Especially the blue ones)

The Post-Braces Party Menu

You're there! You made it! Congratulations!

Celebrations are good. What have you missed the most? Have it in spades now. Do you want to bite your way through a big carrot? Gnaw clean a cob of corn? Chomp into an apple? Munch nuts? Scarf popcorn? Guzzle soda? Make your list. Invite your friends. Enjoy the food. Enjoy the freedom.

Brace yourself for the charming new smile you present the world.

Appendix

The Choice

"Well, my teeth are straighter now."
Lynn

Why do we do it?

Braces can be expensive, time-consuming, uncomfortable, and life-altering. They affect appearance, diet, dining, sex life, and perhaps professional life as well. Yet, according to the American Association of Orthodontists, one out of every five orthodontic patients in this country is an adult. Seventy percent of those are female.

Why do we do it? People opt for braces for these reasons: cosmetics (appearance), malocclusion ("bad bite"), and trauma (damage has been inflicted on the teeth or jaw). The considerations are dental health, function, and psychological well-being.

Cosmetics and Malocclusion

SOUND BITE

Your mouth is a pretty important area. It's [braces are] an easy cosmetic versus other surgeries. You should really smile.
Jeannie

Without the facial asymmetry or the visual imperfections of malocclusion, the cosmetic issue would not exist. We classify as cosmetic those situations that do not risk dental health.

There are three main kinds of malocclusion. "Class I teeth are crowded, crooked, too far apart, or turned at an angle. Class II is usually called an over bite—the upper teeth are too far in front of the lower ones. Class III, the under bite, is the opposite—lower teeth project in front of the upper teeth and jaw." ("A Bit About Bites" by AAO, Robert Johnson and Scholastic, Evan Levine, editor.)

You can inherit or acquire malocclusions. If your problem is extra or missing teeth, crowded teeth, spaces between teeth, or a cleft palate, you probably inherited the malocclusion. But you may have given yourself the malocclusion by sucking your thumb or by thrusting your tongue. Some malocclusions result from dental disease, from the airway being restricted by tonsils and adenoids, or from premature loss of permanent teeth. (AAO pamphlet "Facts About Orthodontics")

The promise of a more beautiful smile motivates many. Most folks want to feel more comfortable smiling, want to stop hiding every time a camera hoves in sight.

SOUND BITE

Such procedures have a troubling tendency to redefine the standards of attractiveness for everyone. As cosmetic medicine and dentistry become more available, all teeth are too crooked, all faces need lifting, all breasts are either too big or too small ... get her the braces if you can afford them.
    Randy Cohen, the Ethicist in The New York Times Magazine (4/25/99)

SOUND BITE

At 35 I saw that the contour of my upper lip was starting to follow those of my very crooked teeth and decided that I didn't want my face to cave in before I was forty. My teeth had collapsed back to their pre-braces look of teenage-hood, and worse. Finally I decided to do it again.
                                        Pam

SOUND BITE

I want to close the gap in my teeth, top front: cosmetically. It's so American. People have nice teeth [here].
                    Angela, from England, living in the USA

Various malocclusion issues aren't critical dental health risks but aren't entirely cosmetic either. For example jumbled teeth can be hard to floss and brush. Straightened teeth eliminate those awkward nooks and crannies where plaque may promote cavities and gum disease so some are motivated to brace themselves by dreams of easier cleaning. Some are motivated to mitigate the stress of misaligned jaws and thus preserve supporting bone and gum tissue.

Others folks brace themselves to improve their bites to rid themselves of TMJ, jaw pain, abnormal wear of tooth surfaces, difficulty chewing, and grinding teeth. Many adults have been through orthodontia before but only had their teeth straightened and did not have their bites properly aligned and so are seeking proper occlusion.

SOUND BITE

Kissing my husband was a little hard. He actually clanked my tooth. Now I never clank. I was having some bone loss and a tooth was loose.
                                                    Jeannie

SOUND BITE

My bite was so far off that I couldn't open wide enough to get a sandwich in my mouth. My jaw would pop each time I opened it.
                                                    Jenny

SOUND BITE

My bite was off. My upper teeth were rubbing against my lower teeth, just like my mother's. Her teeth wore down to the dentine. When I was taking the kids in, I thought I'd ask the dentist about it. He said I had occlusal crowding. Oh yeah. This is classic. He said, "We can make this better." I was under the impression it would take a year or so.

Lynn

SOUND BITE

I had caps put on my front teeth when I was a teenager but they never fit right and were causing the teeth underneath to come loose. I wish I would have known that I had this problem sooner so I could have done something sooner.

Randee

SOUND BITE

My back molars rotated.

Second-time wearer, Lisa

Trauma

Trauma victims may have few choices about

orthodontia. They may need reconstructive work,

requiring braces to stabilize their teeth. Often

prosthodontics succeed better after orthodontics. In the

face of what these individuals must endure, those of us

with cosmetic issues could learn significant lessons about

composure and persistence.

SOUND BITE

*My oral surgeon told me a year after my bike
accident that I would need braces. My braces
were secondary to my surgery. My surgery was
supposed to relocate my jaw, to get my upper and
lower jaws lined up.*
                    JoAnn, bike-accident victim

Thankfully, plastic surgeons and orthodontists are

available if an accident disturbs oral mechanics and

health. They are able to restore us to an esthetic and

functional whole. We are truly appreciative of their

services.